Integrating a Palliative Approach:
ESSENTIALS FOR PERSONAL SUPPORT WORKERS

WORKBOOK

Second Edition, Revised

Katherine Murray

RN, BSN, MA

Life and Death Matters
Victoria, BC

Life & Death Matters

www.lifeanddeathmatters.ca

Published by Life and Death Matters, Victoria, BC, Canada
www.lifeanddeathmatters.ca

Illustrations by Joanne Thomson
Editing by Ann-Marie Gilbert
Design by Greg Glover

ISBN 978-1-926923-17-8 (pbk.)

Disclaimer

This book is intended only as a resource of general education on the subject matter. Every effort has been made to ensure the accuracy of the information it contains; however, there is no guarantee that the information will remain current beyond the date of publication. The information and techniques provided in this book should be used in consultation with qualified medical health professionals and should not be considered a replacement, substitute, or alternative for their guidance, assessment, or treatment. The author and publisher accept no responsibility or liability with respect to any person or entity for loss or damage or any other problem caused or alleged to be caused directly or indirectly by information contained in this book.

Table of Contents

Reflective Writing: A Learning Practice

Our "baggage" is made up of the beliefs and values that each of us has learned and accumulated. Our baggage is reflected every day in our actions and words. In order to effectively meet the needs of dying people, you, as a personal support worker (PSW), must become aware of your own beliefs and values, and learn how to set them aside so they don't interfere with your ability to provide person-centred care. When you become conscious of your beliefs and values, you can acknowledge them without imposing them on others.

Reflective writing is a way to identify and reflect on your own beliefs and values. This workbook will help you begin writing about them in a non-critical way. When you write, ignore spelling, grammar, and anything else that distracts you. Avoid analyzing your writing. Your goal is to freely express yourself. Ignore the critic inside. Include drawings, write in point form or full sentences, and use coloured pens or pencils or anything else that helps you express yourself. You may need to reflect and write several times when thinking through an important topic. This is normal. The awareness that you gain from the writing is more important than what the writing looks like.

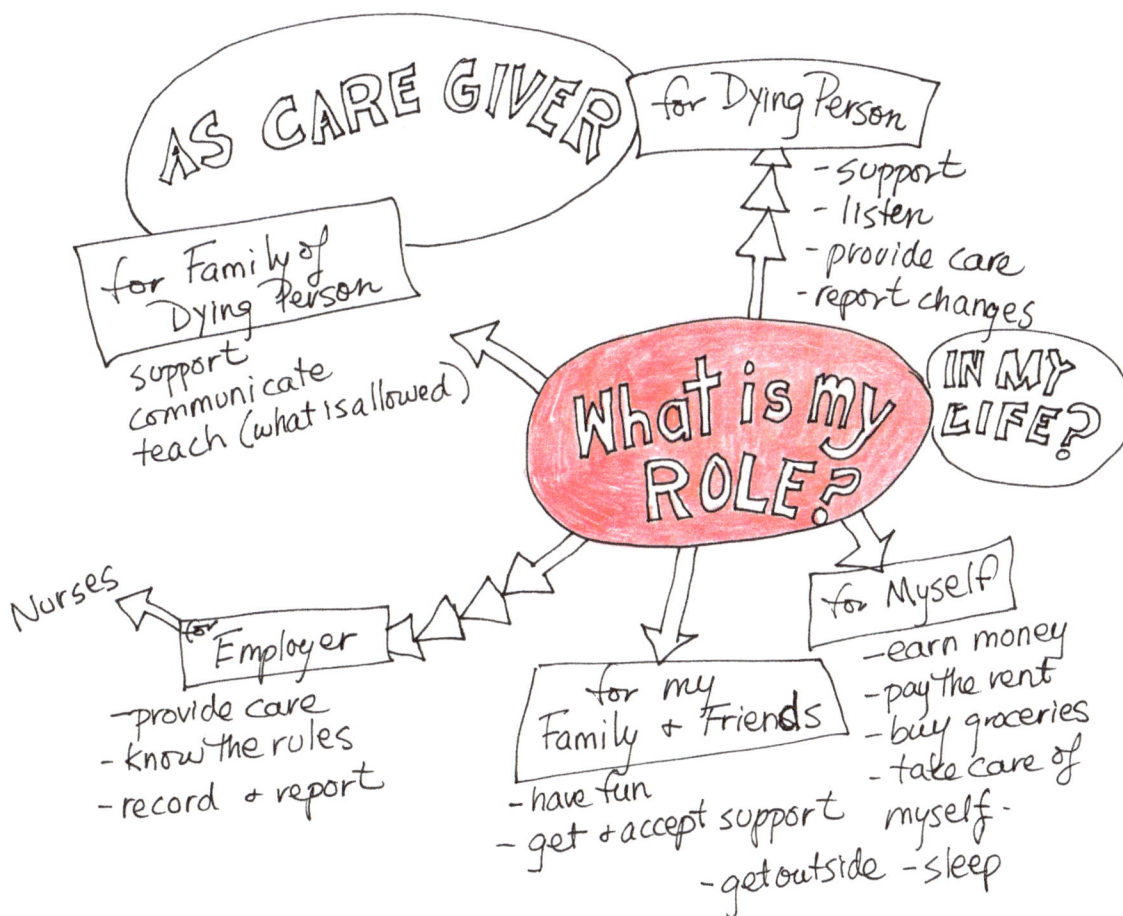

When you feel you have exhausted a topic, take a moment to read what you have written and reflect on it. It is okay to feel surprised, shocked, happy, sad, or any other emotion. These feelings are part of the reflective writing process. If your feelings are particularly strong, you may want to explore them further. This process of writing and reflecting will help you become aware of your own beliefs and values.

Later in the workbook, you are asked to write reflectively. You will be able to identify areas in which your current beliefs may get in the way of caregiving. Once you have identified them, you may want to spend time exploring where the beliefs came from and how they help or interfere with your ability to provide good care.

Choose a quiet and peaceful place for writing. Listen to your inner self, and enter into this practice with an open mind, prepared for self-discovery.

reflections

Understanding Dying and a Palliative Approach

Understanding Your Beliefs and Baggage

1. One key message in the text is that the principles of palliative care can be integrated into care early in the dying process. Is this a new concept for you? Write about this idea. What are the benefits of the palliative approach? Do you already follow some of these principles?

_____

_____

_____

_____

_____

_____

_____

_____

_____

_____

_____

_____

Solidifying Concepts

2a. Identify two key changes in the way that people die differently now than they did 100 years ago.

  i. _____

  ii. _____

2b. Considering the aging population and changes to the way people die, what are two challenges in providing care for dying people now?

  i. _____

  ii. _____

3. Review the common patterns of decline in Chapter 1 of the text. Complete the table below.

Pattern of decline	Impacts on the person	Impacts on the family	Ways that you as a PSW can support the person and the family
Steady decline	1. 2.	1. 2.	1. 2.
Stuttering decline	1. 2.	1. 2.	1. 2.
Slow decline	1. 2.	1. 2.	1. 2.
Sudden death	1. 2.	1. 2.	1. 2.

4. Using the text, define the following terms:

   a. Dementia _____

   b. End of life _____

   c. Holistic care _____

   d. Hospice _____

   e. Palliative care _____

   f. Palliative approach to care _____

5. List the principles of palliative care in your own words.

   _____

   _____

   _____

   _____

   _____

   _____

   _____

   _____

   _____

   _____

   _____

6. Circle the best definition: A "palliative approach" is:

   a. The integration of palliative care principles, practices, and philosophy into care for people with cancer, started in the last six months before death.

   b. The integration of palliative care principles, practices, and philosophy into care for people with all life-limiting illnesses, early in the disease process, across all care settings.

   c. The integration of palliative care principles, practices, and philosophy into care for people with all life-limiting illnesses, for the last six months of life.

7. People are holistic beings, which means that they have

    a. Physical, emotional, and psychosocial needs

    b. Physical, sexual, and spiritual needs

    c. Physical, emotional, psychosocial, sexual and spiritual needs.

    d. Physical, emotional, psychosocial, financial, and spiritual needs

8. Circle the correct answer to indicate whether the following statements are true or false. If a statement is false, provide the reason it is false.

    a. Palliative care regards dying as a natural process, considers the person and family as the unit of care, and continues through death and into bereavement.

    True   False

    _____

    b. Palliative care is active, holistic care exclusively for older individuals with serious health-related suffering due to severe illness.

    True   False

    _____

    c. Palliative care may improve a person's quality of life through the prevention and relief of suffering.

    True   False

    _____

    d. All people with life-limiting conditions can potentially benefit from a palliative approach.

    True   False

    _____

9. What can be learned when an HCP asks the "Surprise Question"?

    _____

    _____

    _____

10. Consider the members of the interdisciplinary health care team who are responsible for care of a person dying in a long-term care facility. In the space below, create a diagram to show the care provided by different members of the interdisciplinary health care team when integrating a palliative approach into a person's care. Use arrows to indicate the flow of information between the team and team members.

11. Care teams can be quite different in urban, rural, or remote areas, and in First Nation, Inuit, or Métis communities. For each location or community listed above, create a diagram to illustrate the different people who are available to be on the care team. Include paid and unpaid people.

Integrating into Practice

12. Working in small groups, consider Figure 7 on page 17 in the text. Using *Tom's Experience—a Stuttering Decline* on page 6. Identify two examples that illustrate how the team followed the principles of palliative care when integrating a palliative approach for Tom and his family..

_____

_____

_____

_____

_____

_____

13. At work or during your practicum, talk with a member of the team and ask who helps to integrate a palliative approach in the care setting, and how to access a specialty palliative care provider when the team is unable to manage the person's symptoms.

14. In the larger group, consider the barriers to accessing and receiving palliative care (page 14 in the text). List the barriers that exist in your community. If time permits, brainstorm ideas for improving access to palliative care for people affected by these barriers..

_____

_____

_____

_____

_____

_____

_____

_____

_____

15. Identify four ways a PSW can integrate a palliative approach into care.

_____

_____

_____

_____

16. In small groups or with a friend or colleague, discuss the following questions:

    a. What is a palliative approach to care?

    b. What is palliative care?

    c. Who is on the care team?

Preparing to Care

Understanding Your Beliefs and Baggage

1. What is self-awareness? Describe it in your own words.

    _____

    _____

    _____

    _____

2. Identify an early experience you had related to death, dying, and/or grief.

    a. Describe the experience.

    _____

    _____

    _____

    _____

    b. What support did you receive? What support would you have liked to receive?

    _____

    _____

    _____

    _____

    c. How did this experience affect you?

    _____

    _____

    _____

    _____

3. Think about the four different patterns (trajectories) of decline, and on the "flip chart" provided draw them in order of your most preferred ("good death") to least preferred ("bad death") way of dying. On the right-hand side of the chart, write two reasons why you placed them in the order you did.

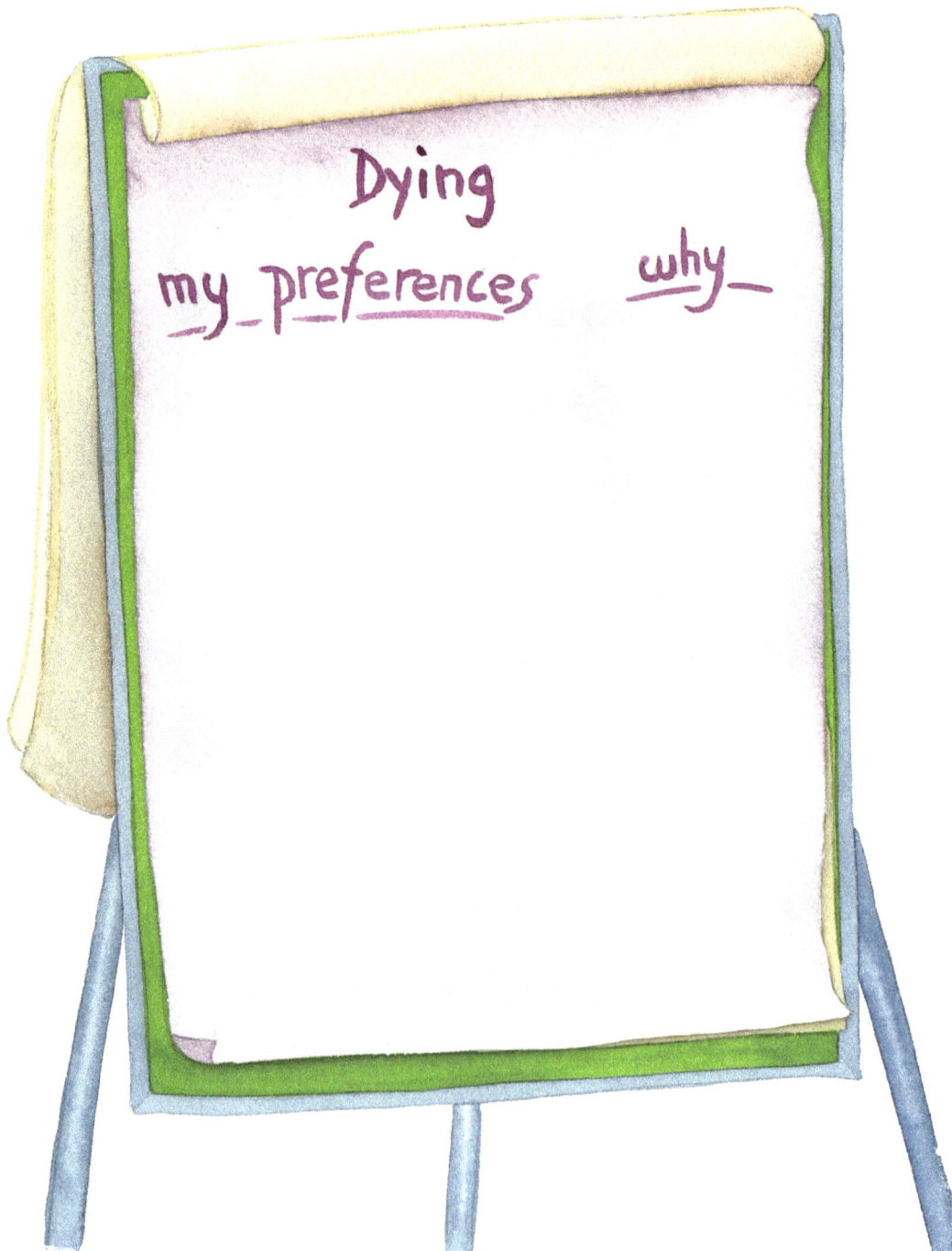

Dying

my preferences   why

4. Reflect on which trajectory or pattern of decline you would hope a loved one would experience when they are dying.

a. Which trajectory would you choose for them?

_____

_____

_____

b. Did you want something different for your loved one than you wanted for yourself? Explain whether you found it harder or easier to imagine and choose a path for someone else instead of for yourself. (Sometimes people have more difficulty making decisions on behalf of another person and may choose more aggressive treatments for someone else than they would want for themselves.)

_____

_____

_____

5. Circle the faces in the illustration below that reflect some of your feelings about working with people who are dying.

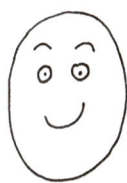 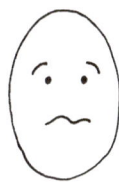 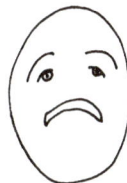 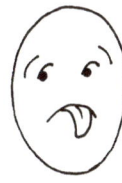 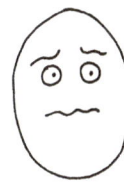 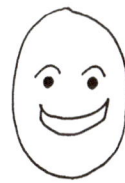

interested   worried   afraid   ill   unsure   eager to learn

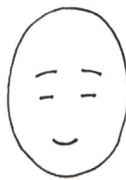 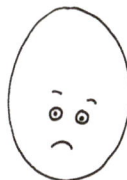 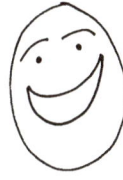 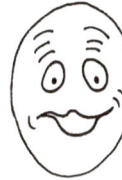 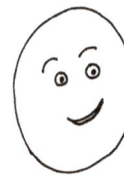 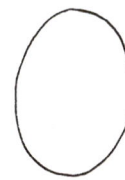

meditative   concerned   glad I can offer support   nervous   honoured   other

6. Label the baggage in the illustration below with some of the beliefs and baggage related to death, dying, and/or grief that you carry with you. What beliefs and baggage will you need to acknowledge and put aside when caring for dying people?

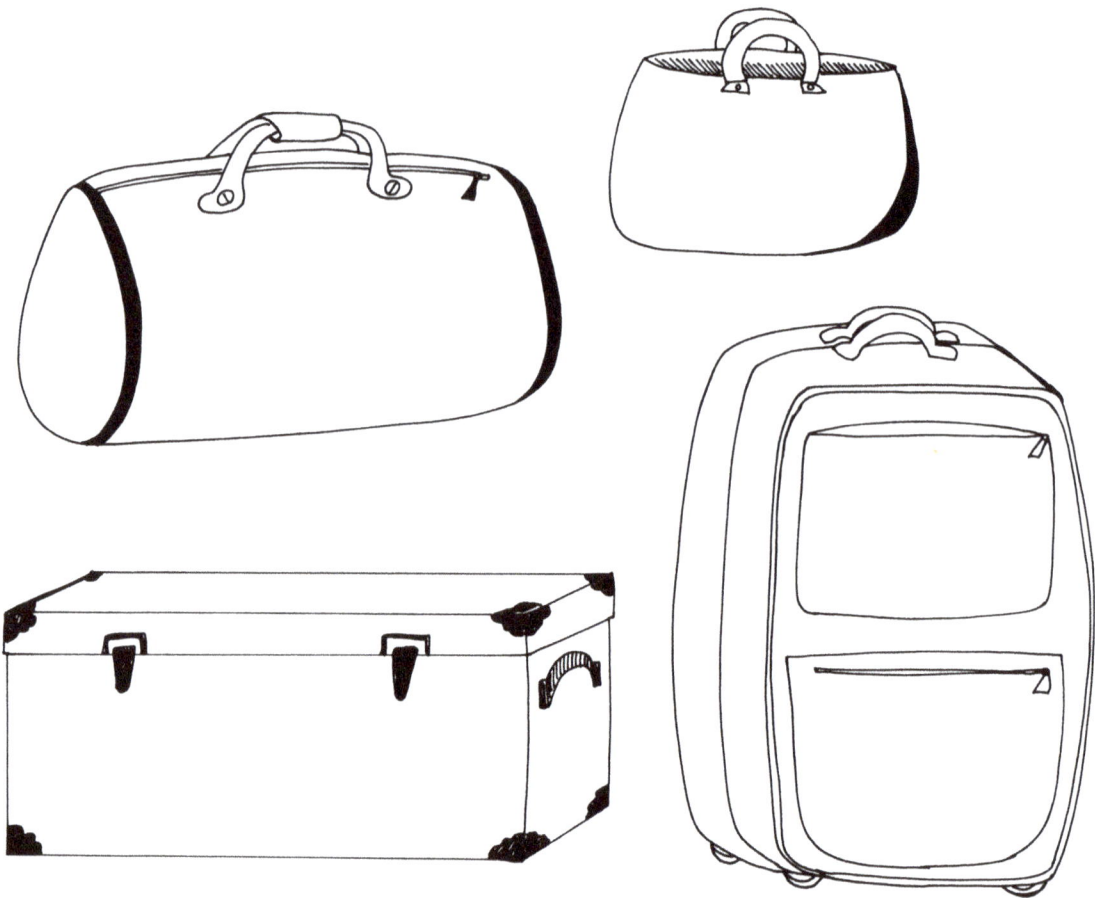

7. Review pages 34 to 40 in Chapter 2 of the text identify best practices and best practice interactions that you use that you use in your life..

_____

_____

_____

_____

_____

_____

_____

8. Recall a time when someone shared a painful experience with you and you wanted to help "fix" the problem. What part of your response suggests that you were in the Fix-It Trap?

_____

_____

_____

_____

9. Answer the reflective questions, listed on page 32 in the text, under the heading "Strategies for addressing systemic bias and racism."

_____

_____

_____

_____

_____

_____

_____

_____

_____

_____

_____

_____

Solidifying Concepts

10. Provide definitions for the following terms:

   a. Culture _____

   _____

   b. Cultural safety _____

   _____

   c. Cultural humility _____

   _____

    d. Cultural sensitivity _____

_____

    e. Cultural awareness _____

_____

    f. Cultural protocols _____

_____

11. As discussed in the "Maintaining Therapeutic Boundaries" section on pages 41 to 45 in the text, therapeutic boundaries are necessary when providing care. Maintaining therapeutic boundaries is not always easy.

    a. How might you know if you are not maintaining boundaries?

        i. _____

        ii. _____

        iii. _____

    b. What steps can you take to establish therapeutic boundaries?

        i. _____

        ii. _____

        iii. _____

12. Review page 38 in the text and provide examples of four common roadblocks to communication.

    a. _____

    b. _____

    c. _____

    d. _____

13. What are the steps to integrating a trauma-informed approach into your practice?

_____

_____

_____

_____

14. Identify whether the following statements express sympathy or empathy (circle your answer):

I feel so sorry for you.	Sympathy	Empathy
I hope you feel better soon.	Sympathy	Empathy
I can hear the sadness in your voice even on the telephone. I am here for you if you want to talk about it.	Sympathy	Empathy
I feel so badly that your mother died.	Sympathy	Empathy
It sounds like you are overwhelmed with things to do. How can I help?	Sympathy	Empathy

15. As a PSW, you help to address the needs of the person and/or their family. Below, circle the activities that PSWs can and should be involved in.

    a. Offer information brochures to the family to clarify services available in your facility.

    b. Share your concerns and observations about the person's level of comfort at their care conference.

    c. Suggest that the family write a list of their concerns, questions, and goals of care to share with the nurse or physician.

    d. Advise the family to increase the person's pain medication.

Integrating into Practice

16. In pairs or small groups, discuss the following:

    a. Similarities and differences between your definitions of self-awareness

    b. Experiences you have had related to death, dying, and/or grief

    c. Feelings you have about working with people who are dying

    d. The concept of baggage that you carry and the need to put baggage aside to care for others.

17. In small groups, describe ways to incorporate the Indigenous Wellness Framework as you are providing care.

18. A vision board is a visualization tool which refers to a board (poster board, cardboard and so on) of any sort used to build a collage of words and pictures that represent your goals and dreams. Create a vision board identifying best practice interactions. For each best practice, identify the skills or behaviours that are already a part of who you are and what you bring naturally to the work. Next, identify best practice skills that you are interested in developing. Work with a colleague or mentor to identify how you can develop those interactions that are not part of who you are into your practice.

19. In small groups, discuss the story about the homeless woman on page 32 in the text. Think about and share an experience you had when you judged someone. Describe the feeling you had about the person. Did your attitude toward them change when you learned more about them? If so, how did it change? What strategies can you use to help you learn not to judge or label people?

20. Work in pairs or small groups to explore one of the Truth and Reconciliation Commission of Canada's Calls to Action identified for health care, summarized on pp. 30–31 of the text. Identify ways PSWs can act on that specific call to action in your community. Share your findings with the larger group.

21. Work in pairs. In the role play described below, one participant will be Person A and the other will be Person B.

    a. Person A talks about a concern or a problem that they have. For example, "I am worried about the exam next week" or "My mom is sick and she may have cancer. My dad is also not well."

    b. Person B will respond with a roadblock to communication (see page 38 in the text).

    c. Person A will consider their internal reaction to this type of response.

    d. Person B will consider how it felt to reply with a roadblock and observe the effect it had on Person A.

    e. Reverse your roles and observe your responses to roadblocks.

    f. Reverse the roles again, but this time ask open-ended questions. Consider how it felt to ask these questions, and how it felt to be asked a question that helped to stimulate thinking, rather than a roadblock.

    g. Discuss your experiences in both roles and compare your feelings when faced with a roadblock versus being asked an open-ended question. Work with your partner to create a list of open-ended questions that encourage communication.

22. It is important that PSWs share information with the team about the person's preferences and goals of care. Reflect on what you would want your family and the team to know about you if they were caring for you when you were dying.

_____

_____

_____

_____

_____

_____

_____

23. Create your own list of characteristics of what would be a good death and a bad death for you.

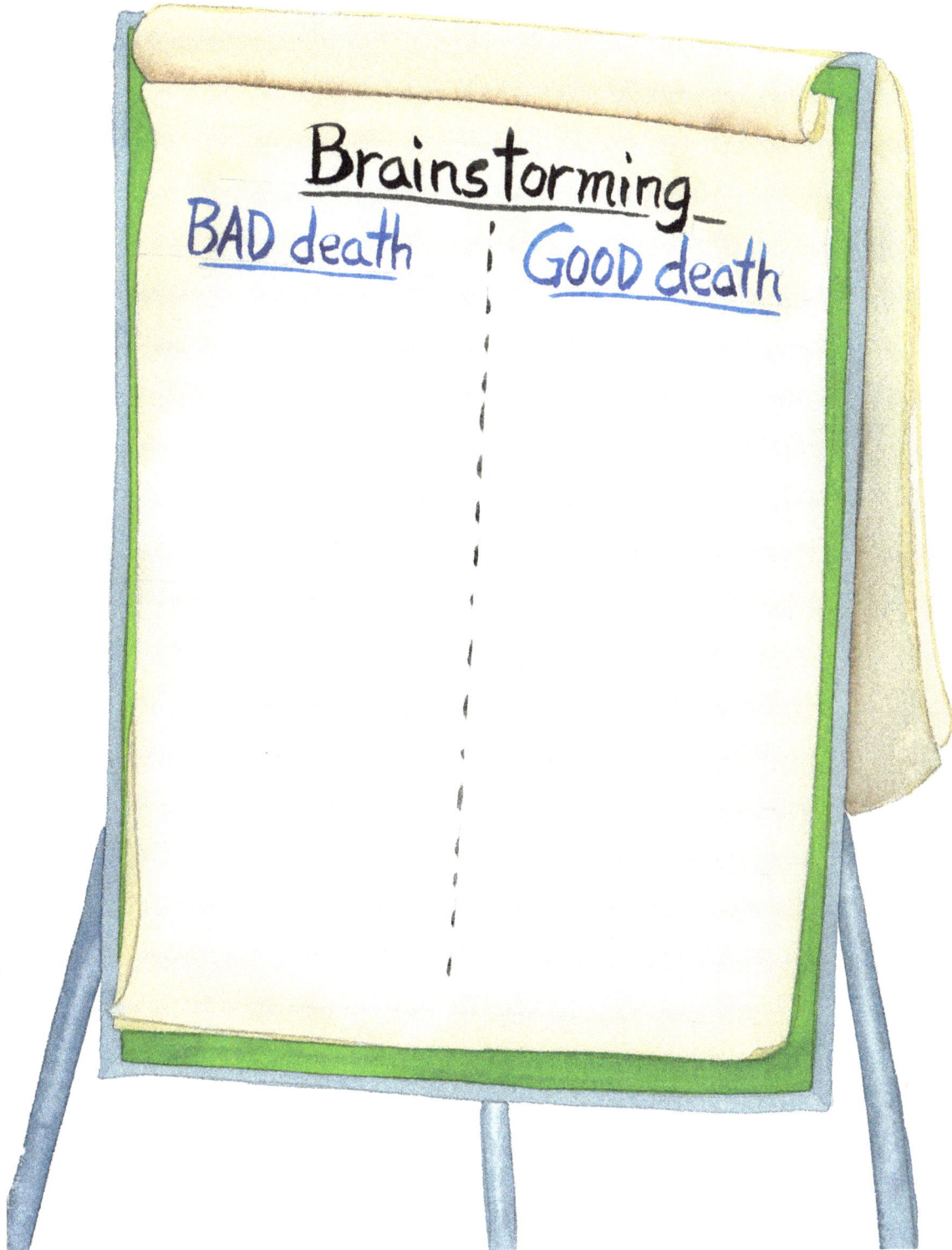

Brainstorming

BAD death	GOOD death

During class or with a partner, compare lists and answer these questions:

a. What characteristics on another person's list surprised you and why?

_____

_____

b. How might you adapt care to help meet individual preferences?

_____

_____

_____

24. Refer to the "Dignity Question" on page 35 in the text. Then imagine that you are dying. What does the team need to know about you to give you the best care possible?

_____

_____

_____

_____

25. Consider the concept of Two-Eyed Seeing on pages 29 and 30 of the text. In the large group, discuss your thoughts about the concept and share ideas on how to integrate this concept into your practice. List two ways to integrate Two-Eyed Seeing into your practice.

_____

_____

_____

_____

26. Systemic bias and racism are present in the health care system.

Option 1: Work in groups to identify people who experience systemic bias and racism in your area. Brainstorm with the group to create a list of practical strategies for combatting systemic bias and racism in your college, workplace, or community. Share your findings with the larger group.

Option 2. Discuss in small groups the unique personal, family, community, and cultural needs that someone will learn when caring for you and your family.

Using Standardized Tools

3

Understanding Your Beliefs and Baggage

1. As a PSW you are a member of the interdisciplinary team. You observe, gather information from the person and the family, and, when needed and as appropriate, you discuss with the team issues that affect the person's quality of life. You collaborate to develop or update the care plan. Reflect on how you feel about collaborating with the team. Write about two strategies you believe will help you to feel more confident in collaborating with the team.

    _____

    _____

    _____

    _____

    _____

    _____

    _____

    _____

    _____

    _____

    _____

Solidifying Concepts

2. Caregivers in many countries and in many settings use the Palliative Performance Scale (PPS) to identify the person's current level of functioning and needs, changes, and the need to adapt the care plan. What five things are measured on the scale?

    a. _____

    b. _____

    c. _____

    d. _____

    e. _____

3. Using words from the PPS, describe a person whose PPS is 20%

_____

_____

_____

4. Using words from the PPS, describe a person whose PPS is 10%.

_____

_____

_____

5. Consider the CSHA Clinical Frailty Scale for the following questions.

   a. What does it mean when a person's frailty value from the CSHA Clinical Frailty Scale increases?

   _____

   b. What might be beneficial for a person when their frailty value is between 4 and 7?

   _____

6. Identify three times to use the Symptom Framework for PSWs?

_____

_____

_____

7. The PAINAD Scale is able to identify if the person is experiencing pain, but is not able to identify the
_____ of the pain.

8. The Psychosocial Assessment Tool helps to identify psychosocial, spiritual, and cultural values and practices of a person. One of the roles of the PSW is to be open and sensitive to values and practices that are different from their own. What are two psychosocial, spiritual or cultural values and practices the care team would need to know about you in order to provide best care possible?

_____

_____

_____

_____

Integrating into Practice

9. Consider the following case. Use the SBAR Communication Tool on page 24 to record information about this person, and then write out what you would report in the space titled "Report."

Eileen is a 98-year-old woman living in her home. She has chronic obstructive pulmonary disease. She receives oxygen through a nasal canula and receives opioids daily to manage her breathlessness. You visit to provide personal care and help her with breakfast.

This morning when you arrived to help her get out of bed, she was frowning and moaning, and she shook her head and said, "No, not today. I'm staying in bed!" You responded, "You are not your usual self. What is happening?" She replied, "My tummy is hurting. I don't want to get up." She suddenly pressed her hands to her midsection, called out in pain, groaned loudly, and rolled onto her side. You asked if a pillow behind her back and between her legs would help make her a bit more comfortable, and when she agreed, you positioned the pillows. Eileen gave you permission to ask her some more questions and talk with the nurse.

She said that the pain in her tummy started this morning. You asked her to point to where it hurts, and she rubbed her hand up and down and back and forth over her abdomen. You asked her to describe the pain, and she replied, "The spasms come and go." You asked her to rate her pain on a scale of 0 to 10, with 10 being the most severe pain that she can imagine and 0 being no pain. She said that when it is bad it is an 8 out of 10, and when it is not bad her abdomen is just tender. She was not able to say how often the pain comes and goes. She thought it may be caused by eating too much dinner. She also did not remember when she had her last bowel movement. She was short of breath as she responded to the questions. You asked how you can best help, and she said she doesn't know, but that she needs something done because the pain is awful. You told her that you will get her some water and will phone the nurse to let her know about the pain, and to ask if she can see Eileen today.

Report _____

_____

_____

_____

_____

_____

10. In classroom discussion or in small groups, discuss the various tools and how they might be used in your community/facility.

_____

_____

S **SITUATION**

My name is _____.

I need to talk with you about _____.

Concern is a   Person's name

- ❑ Change in person's condition
- ❑ Ongoing issue
- ❑ Safety issue
- ❑ Family issue

Is it a good time to talk now? When?

B **BACKGROUND**

They are experiencing [insert symptoms] _____

Relevant information (Include observations from PPS)

A **ASSESSMENT**

Symptom

(Record information gathered with the Symptom Framework for PSWs)

Onset	
Provoking/Palliating	
Quality	
Region/Radiating	
Severity	
Treatment	
Understanding	
Values	
What else?	

Other concerns:

R **REQUEST/RECOMMENDATION**

Can you come and see _____?

What do you recommend that I do now?

What is the plan moving forward?

Supporting Physical Comfort

4

Part 1: Principles and Practices

Understanding Your Beliefs and Baggage

1. Reflect on your experiences of pain and on your family's experiences of pain. Consider your beliefs about pain management. Did you grow up in a home in which family members were comfortable with using medications to manage pain, or do you come from a home in which family members opposed the use of medications? Reflect on and write about this.

_____

_____

_____

_____

_____

_____

_____

2. Reflect on your beliefs about opioids and the use of opioids for managing symptoms. Identify any beliefs, values, or biases that you may hold that will influence how you feel about the person you are caring for receiving opioids.

_____

_____

_____

_____

_____

_____

_____

3. Consider a time when you were ill or experiencing pain. Reflect on what might have helped you to feel more comfortable. What would you like someone to have in their comfort basket if that person were caring for you?

_____

_____

_____

_____

Solidifying Concepts

4. Circle the principles that guide the health care team in supporting physical comfort.

   a. Focus on the person's goals of care.

   b. Individualize comfort measures to meet the needs of the person.

   c. Use medications to manage symptoms only when death is imminent.

   d. Monitor, record, and report the person's responses to medications and other comfort measures.

   e. Provide information and education to help the person and family understand symptom management.

5. Circle the principles that guide the team in making decisions about administration of medications for symptom management.

   a. Comfort measures may help improve comfort.

   b. Medications should be given only after pain occurs, not on a regular schedule.

   c. Breakthrough doses are used when a symptom recurs between regularly scheduled doses.

   d. A combination of medications may be necessary to control a symptom and side effects.

   e. Side effects and fears or concerns about medications should be recorded and reported.

   f. The team determines the goal for pain relief.

6. Opioids are commonly used to help manage pain and difficulty breathing.

   True   False   (circle your answer)

7. These are the four most common side effects of opioids (circle your answer):

   a. Nausea/vomiting, drowsiness, addiction, confusion

   b. Nausea/vomiting, drowsiness, confusion, insomnia

   c. Constipation, addiction, nausea/vomiting, confusion

   d. Nausea/vomiting, constipation, drowsiness, confusion

8. Describe each of the four common fears and misunderstandings about using opioids for symptom management.

   a. _____

   _____

   b. _____

   _____

   c. _____

   _____

   d. _____

   _____

9. Why is it important to provide medications for symptom management regularly, around the clock?

   _____

   _____

   _____

   _____

10. Two common side effects of opioids are drowsiness and constipation.

    True   **False**   (circle your answer)

11. What would be the consequences of not providing medications (e.g., opioids) regularly for a person experiencing pain?

_____

_____

_____

12. Traditional healing and medicines benefit the person spiritually, emotionally, and culturally. How can you prepare so that a person feels comfortable requesting and accessing traditional medicine and healing practices?

a. _____

b. _____

c. _____

d. _____

e. _____

13. List the reasons why a person might benefit from the inclusion of complementary and alternative therapies in their care.

a. _____

b. _____

c. _____

Part 2: Common Symptoms

Anorexia and Cachexia

Understanding Your Beliefs and Baggage

14. Read "Profound Truths of Nutrition" on page 100 in the text. Reflect on how you feel when reading these truths. Discuss the truths as a class or in small groups.

_____

_____

_____

_____

_____

_____

_____

_____

_____

_____

Solidifying Concepts

15. A dying person often loses weight and loses interest in eating. Refer to the story about Yetta's experience on page 4 in the text.

a. What did Yetta do to address her lack of appetite?

_____

_____

b. Identify four things that a PSW can do to help a person experiencing decrease in appetite.

i. _____

ii. _____

iii. _____

iv. _____

v. _____

16. Identify three ways that you and the team can support the family of a person experiencing anorexia and cachexia.

_____

_____

_____

_____

_____

_____

_____

For the questions related to symptoms, refer to the relevant topic area in the text and the Symptom Framework for PSWs to complete the tables

Changes in Bowel and Bladder Function

Solidifying Concepts

17. List two strategies to help prevent constipation in a person with limited mobility.

a. _____

b. _____

18. Use pages 102 to 104 of the text to complete the table below.

What you might observe if a person is constipated	What you might ask the person to better understand their needs	Comfort measures that might be helpful	Ways to support family
1.	1.	1.	1.
2.	2.	2.	2.
3.	3.	3.	3.

Dehydration

Solidifying Concepts

19. Read pages 104 to 106 in the text to complete the table below.

What you might observe if a person is dehydrated	What you might ask the person to better understand their needs	Comfort measures that might be helpful	Ways to support family
1.	1.	1.	1.
2.	2.	2.	2.
3.	3.	3.	3.

Delirium

Solidifying Concepts

20.

Mrs. Marsh is a resident at your facility. You are called by Mrs. Marsh's daughter, who is concerned about her mother's recent behaviour changes, including pacing, confusion, inability to carry on a conversation, and refusing to take medication.

Complete the table below using the case provided and information from pages 108 to 114 of the text.

What you might observe if a person has delirium	What you might ask the person to better understand their needs	Comfort measures that might be helpful	Ways to support family
1.	1.	1.	1.
2.	2.	2.	2.
3.	3.	3.	3.

21. Indicate in the following table the differences between dementia and delirium.

	Delirium	Dementia
Causes		
Time frame of onset		
Brain changes—permanent or reversible?		
Caused by body changes (yes/no)		
Presence of anxiety, fear, or paranoia		

Integrating into Practice

22.

You are providing care for an Indigenous person in their home in an isolated community. There is no physician or nurse available to visit. The health care team supports you through phone calls. The person is experiencing delirium. You know that the family wants to keep their loved one in the community and does not want to transfer them to the hospital, which is a four-hour drive away. You need to call the nurse or physician to update them on the changes, and to develop a care plan that will meet the needs and the goals of the person, family, and community members who are caring for the person. You know that you need to gather information by observing and interacting with the person. You also know that you will need to talk with the family and the community members who are involved to understand their needs and their desire to keep the person at home.

Identify three tools that will help you gather information and share information about the person, their delirium, the family and their needs/wishes.

_____

_____

_____

Difficult Breathing

Understanding Your Beliefs and Baggage

23. Complete the exercise below to experience difficult breathing (dyspnea).

Dyspnea Exercise

Materials: A drinking straw

Location: A place with room to walk

Note: People with respiratory or heart problems should not participate in this exercise.

Exercise

   a. Pinch your nostrils to cut off airflow through them.

   b. Place the straw in your mouth and begin breathing through it.

   c. Walk around for two minutes.

   d. At the end of two minutes, remove the straw from your mouth and stop plugging your nose. Take a moment to allow your breathing and sensations to return to normal.

You have just experienced sensations similar to those that people with dyspnea have.

Answer the following questions:

24. What did the experience feel like? Describe it.

_____

_____

_____

25. What were your thoughts as the exercise progressed?

_____

_____

_____

26. How do feel you would respond if that sensation happened to you suddenly? What would you think was happening?

_____

_____

_____

Solidifying Concepts

27. Complete the table below using pages 117 to 120 of the text.

How you might prevent difficulty with breathing	What you might observe if a person has difficulty with breathing	What you might ask a dying person to better understand their needs	Comfort measures that might be helpful
1.	1.	1.	1.
2.	2.	2.	2.
3.	3.	3.	3.

Fatigue

Solidifying Concepts

28. If the person you are caring for has a PPS of 40% and is very fatigued, what comfort strategies can you suggest that might help them have the energy to accomplish their priority activities? Complete the table below using pages 121 to 123 of the text.

How you might prevent fatigue	What you might ask the person to better understand their needs	Comfort measures that might be helpful
1.	1.	1.
2.	2.	2.
3.	3.	3.

Mouth Discomfort

Solidifying Concepts

29. Complete the table below with information from pages 124 to 127 of the text.

What you might observe if a person has a dry mouth	What you might ask a person to better understand their needs	Comfort measures that might be helpful
1.	1.	1.
2.	2.	2.
3.	3.	3.

Nausea and Vomiting

Solidifying Concepts

30. Consider this scenario.

> She was crying on the bed when I entered her room.
>
> She said, "I'm so tired of this nausea; I wish I could just die."
>
> I sat with her and held her hand. It was the only way I thought I could be helpful at that moment.
>
> When she was less distressed, we talked. I used the Symptom Framework for PSWs to better understand what was happening, and then I phoned the nurse to report.

a. Remember a time when you or a friend or family member were nauseated. Using the Symptom Framework for PSWs adapted for nausea and vomiting on page 37, consider possible answers that a nauseous person might give you when you ask the questions. Write what you "heard" as though you were recording for a person experiencing nausea.

Symptom Framework adapted for nausea and vomiting

O	**Onset**	When did the symptom begin? Is this new, or has this happened before? Did it start suddenly or slowly?
P	**Provoking/Palliating**	What makes the symptom feel better? Worse?
Q	**Quality**	Can you describe the discomfort? How does this symptom affect you?
R	**Region/Radiating**	Where are you feeling the symptom?
S	**Severity**	How severe is the symptom? 0 = no symptom and 10 = the worst imaginable Small, medium, large Mild, moderate, severe
T	**Treatment**	What do you think might be helpful?
U	**Understanding**	What do you think might be happening?
V	**Values**	What are your goals for the symptom?
W	**What else?**	What else do you want me to know or do? **For the PSW:** Consider your knowledge of this person—what do you see? What do you believe would be helpful?

b. Using the SBAR Communication Tool and the notes you wrote about the previous scenario, write out the verbal report you would provide to the nurse.

S

SITUATION
My name is _____.
I need to talk with you about _____.
Concern is a   Person's name
    ❏ Change in person's condition
    ❏ Ongoing issue
    ❏ Safety issue
    ❏ Family issue
Is it a good time to talk now? When?

B

BACKGROUND
They are experiencing nausea and vomiting.
Relevant information (Include observations from PPS)

A

ASSESSMENT
Symptom
(Record information gathered with the Symptom Framework for PSWs)

Onset	
Provoking/Palliating	
Quality	
Region/Radiating	
Severity	
Treatment	
Understanding	
Values	
What else?	

Other concerns:

R

REQUEST/RECOMMENDATION
Can you come and see _____?
What do you recommend that I do now?
What is the plan moving forward?

Pain

Integrating into Practice

Role-Plays

Questions 31 and 32 are role-play exercises. Two role-plays are included so that each student can participate in at least one role-play as the PSW.

    a. Identify your group (either two or three people) for the role-play exercises.

    b. Decide who will play each role for each of the role-plays. The PSW part must be played by different students for Q 31 and 32.

    c. Fill in the role assignments for each role-play in the space provided below.

    d. Role descriptions are provided for each role in both role-plays. Read ONLY the description for your role assignment in each role-play.

31. Role Assignments for Mr. J's Pain

PSW _____ **Mr. J** _____ **Nurse Supervisor** _____

(If working in pairs, the instructor can play the part of the nurse supervisor).

Role Descriptions
PSW: The description of your role appears in the box on the following page. Use the Symptom Framework for PSWs adapted for pain on page 69 and the SBAR tools provided on page 70. Answer Q 31 a, b, c, and d on page 41.
Mr. J and **Nurse Supervisor**: page 42.

Goals: In this roleplay you will:

- Demonstrate how to gather information using the Symptom Framework for PSWs, adapted for pain (page 69).

- Demonstrate how to record and report information in a phone call with the nurse using the SBAR communication tool (page 70).

Background

Mr. J is a 75-year-old male who lives alone. He has prostate cancer and is dying. You visit Mr. J in his home daily to assist him with personal care, remind him to take his medications and set out a meal. Usually, Mr. J is happy to see you and he loves to talk with you.

Current Scenario

When you enter his home today, you notice his dinner from last night is still on the table and the food appears untouched. Mr. J appears to be frowning and scowling and does not look like his usual pleasant self this morning. When you greet him, he mumbles a response. You ask him how he is doing, and he tells you that he did not sleep last night, is in pain, and can hardly move because his left hip is so sore. He says he is tired of being sick. When you suggest a bath, he says that there is no way that he can even get to the bathroom.

You realize Mr. J's condition has changed and that you need to gather and record information about his pain and report it to the nurse promptly. You remember that you can use the System Framework for PSWs adapted for pain to gather information.

Proceed with gathering information about Mr. J's pain and then prepare a report using the SBAR communication tool for the nurse supervisor.

Mr. J. is able to answer all of your questions. Complete the following:

a. Gather information about Mr. J's pain using the Symptom Framework for PSWs adapted for pain.

b. Record your observations in Mr. J's "chart" (below).

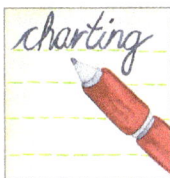

_____

_____

_____

_____

_____

_____

_____

_____

_____

_____

c. Use the SBAR tool to prepare an oral report. Deliver the oral report to the nurse.

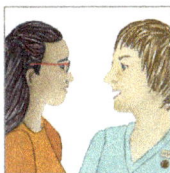

_____

_____

_____

_____

_____

_____

_____

_____

_____

_____

_____

d. Discuss what you learned in this exercise with your role-play partner.

PATIENT'S ROLE – MR. J

Goal: To roleplay the part of Mr. J, using this summary to guide your responses to the PSW.

Do not provide information if the PSW does not ask for it.

A PSW comes to see you every day. Usually, you are pleasant and talkative, but today you are quieter, gritting your teeth and frowning. You are in a lot of pain and need help. The pain started yesterday after you fell on the way to the kitchen. You tripped over the edge of an area rug on the floor. Thankfully your neighbour was there and helped you back to bed. You figure that you hurt your hip when you fell; it has been aching ever since and will not stop. It is the worst pain you have had since getting sick and is almost as bad as when you broke your leg 20 years ago.

The pain medications that you usually take five times a day help a little, but only for an hour or so. Your neighbour gave you a cold pack, but you can't get out of bed to get it. Rubbing your hip helps a bit.

When asked, you rate your pain at 7 on a scale where 0 is no pain and 10 is the worst pain you can imagine. Moving your leg makes the pain worse. You couldn't sleep last night and are feeling exhausted. You are miserable from the pain but glad the PSW is there because you need help.

NURSE SUPERVISOR'S ROLE – MR. J

Goal: To receive the report on Mr. J from the PSW and ask questions if needed.

The role of the nurse can be played by the instructor or by the third student. Listen to the PSW's report while looking at the Symptom Framework for PSWs adapted for pain and the SBAR communication tool. Ask questions to fill in any gaps in the information provided. Thank the PSW and let them know that you will be over to assess Mr. J in about 30 minutes.

32. Role Assignments for Mr. W's Pain

PSW _____ Mr. W _____ Nurse Supervisor _____

(If working in pairs, the instructor can play the part of the nurse supervisor).

Role Descriptions
PSW: The description of your role appears in the box below. Use the Symptom Framework for PSWs adapted for pain on page 69 and the SBAR tools provided on page 70. Answer Q 32 a, b, c, and d on page 44.

Mr. J and **Nurse Supervisor**: page 45.

PSW's ROLE – MR. W

Goals: In this roleplay you will:

- Demonstrate how to gather information using the Symptom Framework for PSWs, adapted for pain (page 69).

- Demonstrate how to record and report information to the nurse in a phone call, using the SBAR communication tool (page 70).

Background

Mr. W is an 85-year-old male that has lived in the long-term care home where you work for two years. He has osteoporosis and a history of multiple fractures. Mr. W. is cognitively able and alert but is frail and slow-moving.

Current Scenario

As you are supporting Mr. W to stand up, he seems hesitant to move and gets out of bed very carefully. When you comment on his slow movements and his apparent stiffness, he says that he is in pain and that can hardly move because his back is so sore. He says he did not sleep much last night. Mr. W is willing to sit in the chair by the bed but does not want to go to the dining room for breakfast. He is very worried about his back.

You realize Mr. W's condition has changed and that you need to gather information, record your observations of his pain, and report to the nurse promptly. You remember that you can use the System Framework for PSWs adapted for pain to gather information. Please proceed with assessing Mr. W's pain and then prepare a report using the SBAR communication tool for the nurse supervisor.

Mr. W. is able to answer all of your questions. Complete the following:

a. Gather information about Mr. W's pain using the Symptom Framework for PSWs on adapted for pain.

b. Record your observations in Mr. W's "chart" (below).

charting

_____

_____

_____

_____

_____

_____

_____

_____

_____

_____

c. Use the SBAR tool to prepare an oral report. Deliver the oral report to the nurse.

_____

_____

_____

_____

_____

_____

_____

_____

_____

_____

_____

d. Discuss what you learned in this exercise with your role-play partner.

Goal: To roleplay the part of Mr. W, using this summary to guide your responses to the PSW.

Do not provide information if the PSW does not ask for it.

The PSW comes to help you get out of bed today. You wish the PSW would take care of everyone else first because you are so sore! Your back hurts worse than it has for ages.

When the PSW asks you questions about your pain, provide the information as described below.

You always have a little bit of back pain, however last night the pain really increased after you went to bed. You don't know what happened to cause it to get so bad. You are worried that you have another fracture and hope the doctor will come see you and check it out.

The pain is worse than the other pains you have had before. This one is terrible! In fact, if they ask you to rate the pain, you might even say this pain rates 8 out of 10 on a scale where 0 is no pain and 10 is the worst pain you can imagine. It hurts in your upper and lower back, and the sharp and shooting pain goes down your legs. It gets worse when you move, and you haven't found anything to make it feel better yet.

You take only the regular medications that the nurse gives you every day at breakfast, lunch and supper. You wish your wife were alive, because she would help you by giving you a warm flannel blanket. You wish you could just stay in bed and not get up, and you definitely do not want to go to breakfast.

NURSE SUPERVISOR'S ROLE – MR. W

Goal: To receive the report on Mr. W from the PSW and ask questions of the PSW as needed.

The role of the nurse can be played by the instructor or by the third student. Listen to the PSW's report while looking at the Symptom Framework for PSWs adapted for pain and the SBAR communication tool. Ask questions to fill in any gaps in the information provided. Thank the PSW and let them know that you will go into Mr. W's room right away to assess him.

33. Refer to the story about Annette on page 134 in the text.

a. How did the PSW identify Annette's pain?

_____

_____

_____

b. What did the PSW do to help address Annette's pain?

_____

_____

_____

c. Write a verbal report to share information with the nurse about Annette.

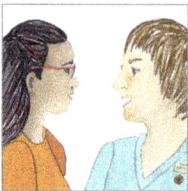

_____

_____

_____

_____

_____

_____

d. Follow-up after giving medication is as important as the original charting to report pain. Write a sample chart entry following up on Annette.

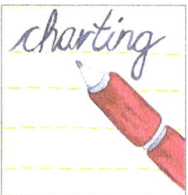

_____

_____

_____

_____

_____

_____

_____

Providing Psychosocial Care

5

Understanding Your Beliefs and Baggage

1. This exercise is designed to help you understand the importance of helping people with life-limiting illnesses determine their priorities and maintain their choices.

   a. In the large box below, list the things that are important to you in your life (e.g., people, activities, events, foods).

   b. In the medium-sized box, write about what you would do if you had only three months to live.

   c. In the small circle, write about what you would do if you had only three days to live.

a

b

c

Note: If you are feeling vulnerable and think that this exercise will be too much for you, work with a colleague or the instructor to adapt this activity to meet your needs. If this exercise triggers strong responses, consider debriefing with a colleague or the instructor.

Now think about your responses to the exercise and do some reflective writing guided by the questions below:

d. What were your feelings as you wrote in the large box? The medium box? The small circle? What thoughts do you associate with these feelings?

_____

_____

_____

_____

_____

_____

e. Write about your decision-making process for what to write in the shapes. How did the items differ as you moved to smaller shapes? How did you decide what to include in the small circle?

_____

_____

_____

_____

_____

_____

f. How would you feel if you were not able or not allowed to do what you identified in the circle? Consider how dying during the COVID-19 pandemic affected the ability of the person to do what they wanted in their last weeks and days and hours. If you had been dying and unable to see family or friends in the last days, how would that be for you? What might have been helpful?

_____

_____

_____

_____

_____

_____

2. Reflect on this story and answer the questions below it.

You have been assisting a person with their personal care regularly for several months. You have become very fond of them and their partner and enjoy providing care. When you arrive today, the partner informs you that the person has decided not to continue with kidney dialysis. The doctors suggest that without dialysis they might have a few weeks to live. You realize that this will shorten their life significantly.

a. What feelings, thoughts, and questions might you have?

_____

_____

_____

b. With whom is it appropriate to discuss your questions and feelings?

_____

_____

c. If you do not agree with the person's choice to discontinue dialysis, what best practice interactions can help you withhold judgment and show respect?

_____

_____

_____

_____

_____

d. What might you say to or do for the person and the partner to show compassion?

_____

_____

_____

_____

_____

Solidifying Concepts

3. Describe why psychosocial care is an essential part of holistic care.

_____

_____

_____

_____

_____

4. Describe what you can do to support a person through transitions when their disease is advancing and the person has been told that a cure is not possible.

_____

_____

_____

_____

_____

_____

5. Identify four key points about dying with dementia.

a. _____

_____

b. _____

_____

c. _____

_____

d. _____

_____

6.

You are caring for a person whose culture is different from yours. The person has just been admitted to your facility. The person's health has declined recently and they are dying imminently. The team needs to talk with the family to provide an update and prepare them for the person's imminent death.

What principles of providing culturally safe care will help you and the team share information in a most helpful and supportive way?

_____

_____

_____

_____

_____

_____

_____

_____

_____

_____

7. As a PSW you support a person's psychosocial needs when you:

a. _____

b. _____

c. _____

d. _____

e. _____

8. List three formal assessment processes that the physician, nurse and social worker might use to gather information about a person's values, beliefs and preferences for care.

a. _____

b. _____

c. _____

9. Identify eight ways that PSWs can support advance care planning.

a. _____

b. _____

c. _____

d. _____

e. _____

f. _____

g. _____

h. _____

10. As a PSW you can advise patients on legal matters and care decisions.

True   False   (circle your answer)

11. Write five things you learned about grief that you did not know before reading the text.

a. _____

b. _____

c. _____

d. _____

e. _____

12. Describe ways to support children whose loved one is dying.

a. _____

_____

b. _____

_____

c. _____

_____

d. _____

_____

Integrating into Practice

13. Complete the exercise below to learn about your personal responses to loss.

Multiple Losses Exercise

On each of six pieces of paper, write down one activity that you enjoy (writing lightly with the pencil will decrease the chance of the writing being legible from the reverse side of the paper when it is turned over). Lay the papers writing side down on the table in front of you. Shuffle them around such that you no longer know which is which. Line them up in a row.

Turn over the middle two pieces of paper and imagine that because of declining health you are no longer able to do these activities. What is your immediate response to having these two activities removed from your life? What do you feel? What do you think?

_____

_____

_____

Resist the urge to change an activity that you lost to a different one. This exercise is designed to help you imagine the multiple losses that dying people experience.

Now imagine it is two weeks later and the doctor tells you that you should no longer do two more of the activities. What do you feel about these new losses? Do you feel better knowing that you still have two activities left?

_____

_____

_____

Now imagine that you wake one morning a month later and are unable to do the remaining two activities. What do you feel? What do you want to do or say?

_____

_____

_____

Discuss your experience with a colleague.

---

14. In small groups, discuss ways to support a person's relationships with their family and community. Include options for a person who is not able to be with their home community, family or culture.

15. Review pages 166 to 167 in the text about grief being a whole-person experience.

a. Mark the illustration below using words, colours, and shapes to indicate how you experience grief and how it affects you physically, emotionally, spiritually, and socially.

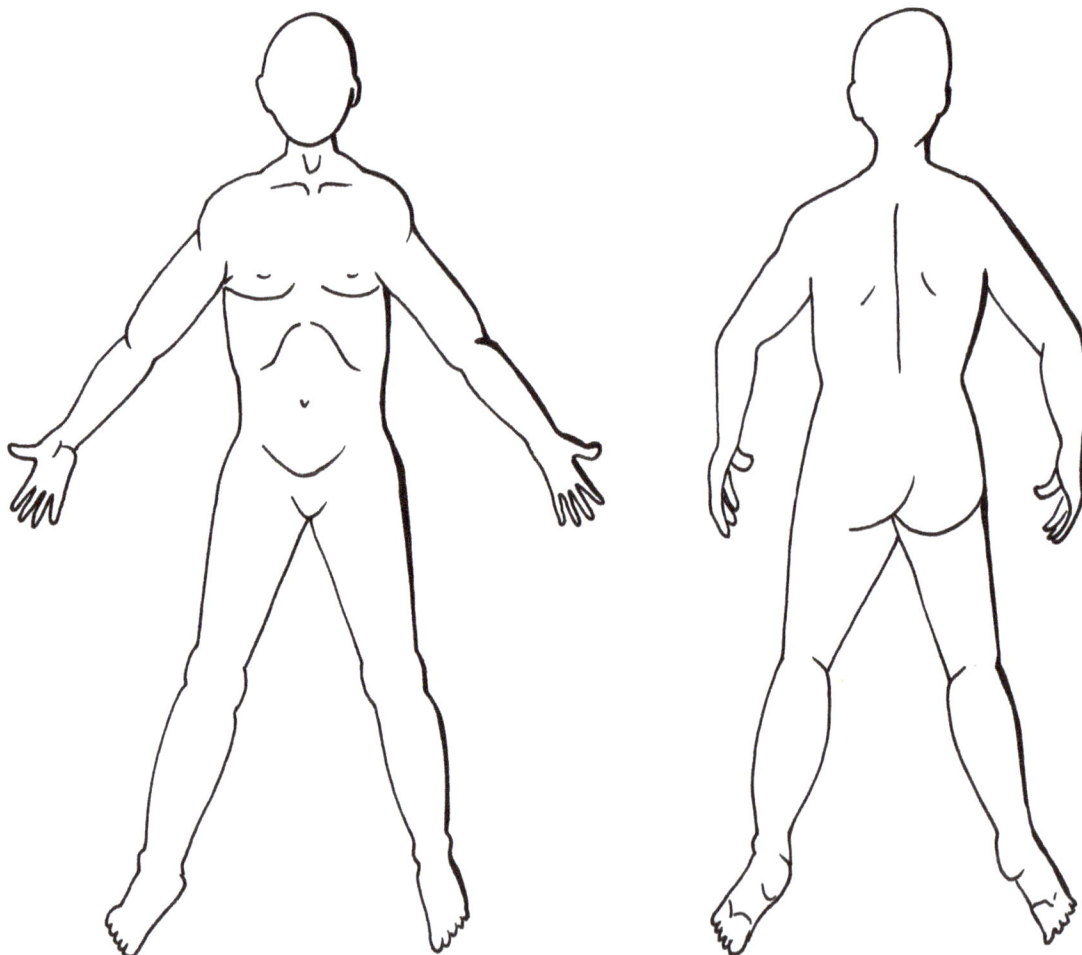

b. Reflect on how grief is a whole person experience.

_____

_____

_____

_____

_____

_____

c. Think about a friend or family member who has experienced loss and grief in their life. Use the illustration below to create a picture of grief as you saw your friend or family member experience it.

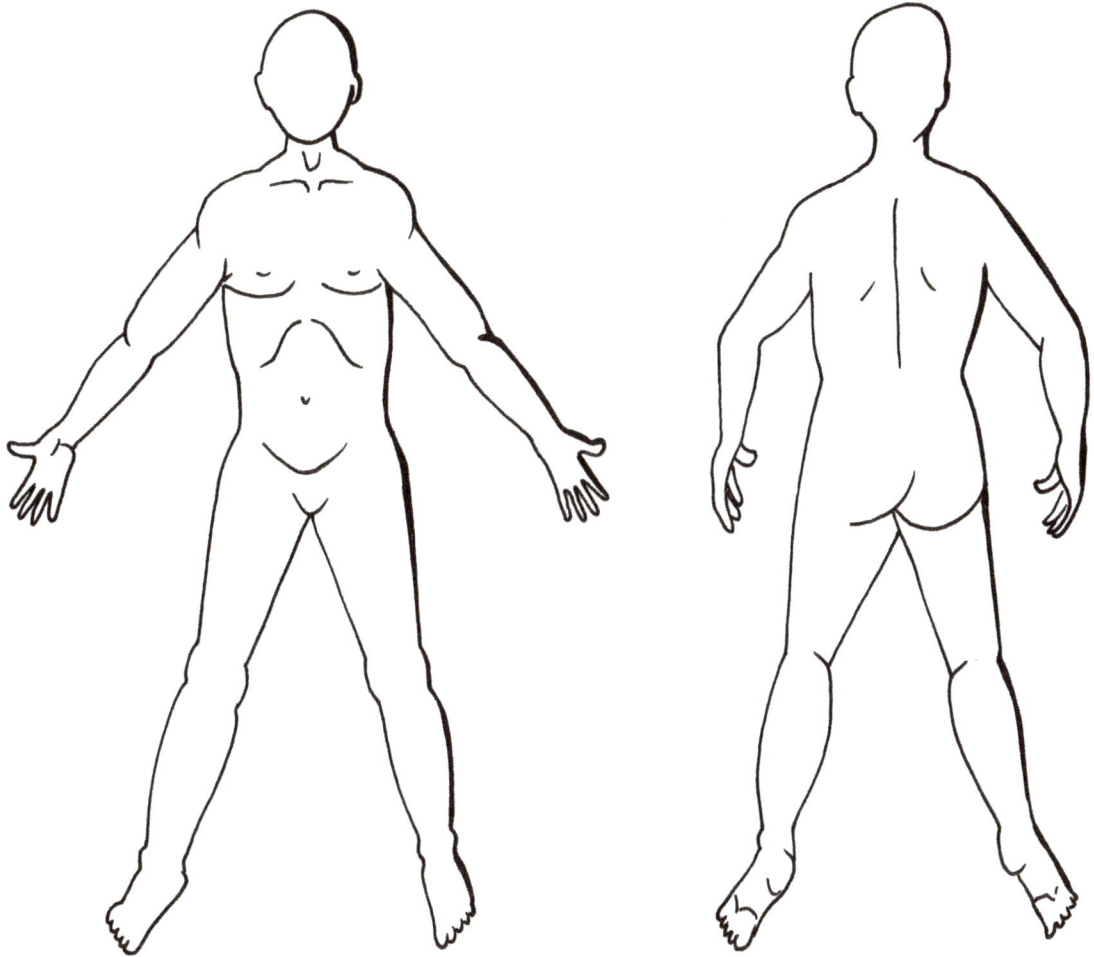

16. Reflect on the ways to support a grieving person (pages 170 to 173). In small groups or independently, list ways that you might support a grieving person.

_____

_____

_____

_____

_____

_____

_____

17. Complete the reflective activity on Medical Assistance in Dying (MAID) on page 162. Then work in pairs or small groups to share your experiences. Acknowledge the different views of your colleagues. Identify follow-up actions for yourself.

_____

_____

_____

_____

_____

_____

_____

_____

_____

_____

_____

_____

_____

_____

_____

_____

_____

_____

_____

_____

_____

_____

Caring in the Last Days and Hours

Understanding Your Beliefs and Baggage

1. Reflect on and write about your feelings regarding caring for someone in their last days and hours and at the time of death. Compare this reflection to the feelings you identified, in exercise 5 and 6 in Chapter 2 of this workbook, about working with people who are dying. Your feelings today may be similar to those you identified before or may have changed.

_____

_____

_____

_____

_____

_____

_____

_____

2. PSWs often provide care for a person's body after death has occurred. For some people this is a sacred ritual; others are not comfortable doing this. Reflect on how you feel about caring for the body after death. If you feel uncomfortable, consider asking a colleague or supervisor to mentor you and help you become more comfortable. You may want to ask for additional opportunities at work to gain experience providing care for the body. Reflect on and write about caring for the body after death.

_____

_____

_____

_____

_____

_____

_____

Solidifying Concepts

3. Refer to pages 186 to 193 in the text and complete the following chart.

Physical changes in the last days and hours	Comfort measures for the dying person	Comfort measures for the family
Decreased physical strength and increased drowsiness		
Reduced intake and difficulty swallowing		
Delirium or confusion		
Agitation or restlessness		
Unresponsiveness		
Irregular breathing		
Congested breathing		
Changes in skin colour and temperature		
Dry eyes		
Decreased urinary output		
Bowel or bladder incontinence		

4. Identify three things the team can do to prepare to provide best care in the last days and hours.

   a. _____

   b. _____

   c. _____

5. The family asks you, "What changes can I expect in the last days and hours?" What are four appropriate ways for you as a PSW to respond?

   a. _____

   b. _____

   c. _____

   d. _____

6. Identify four signs that indicate that the person has died.

   _____

   _____

   _____

   _____

7. List 5 tasks to be completed in caring for the body following death.

   _____

   _____

   _____

   _____

   _____

8. It is always important to know what a person's DNR status is before entering their home.

   True   False   (circle your answer)

9. Describe three ways you can support the family after the death of their loved one. (See pages 198–199.)

a. _____

_____

b. _____

_____

c. _____

_____

10. List three ways you can you show respect and support for people whose cultural traditions or spiritual practices are different from yours.

a. _____

b. _____

c. _____

11. Review page 202 in the text and fill in the blanks in the paragraph below.

When a person's death is sudden, unexpected, or occurs within 24 hours of admission to a hospital, the coroner is notified. The role of the coroner is to confirm the _____ of the person who died and the probable _____ and _____ of death. The coroner classifies the death as natural, accidental, suicide, homicide, or undetermined.

Integrating into Practice

12. Describe two reasons why it is important to explore the family's understanding when they are asking how long the person might live.

a. _____

_____

b. _____

_____

13. Discuss the topics below in small groups or with a colleague.

    a. Supporting a family whose traditions and practices in caring for the body after death are different from what you know

    b. Ways to support the family when they participate in a cultural practice that does not have meaning for you or seems unnecessary

14. Reflect on the following scenario:

You have been providing care for an Indigenous person (or a person from a culture different from yours) for almost seven months, and they are nearing their last days and hours. Because the family knows you and is comfortable with you, they ask you to find space for rituals and traditional ceremonies, and for many members of the community to meet as the person dies and after death.

In small groups, discuss how you would respond to this request in a culturally safe manner. Consider different care locations (e.g., long-term care, acute care, hospice, home), and brainstorm ways to create space and privacy in these locations for the person, their family, and their community as they provide rituals and ceremonies for their dying loved one. If you do not have personal experience in these locations, ask your instructor to provide a brief overview of the different caregiving spaces in your community.

Meet with the larger group and share your ideas for providing space.

15. When you are at work or during a practicum, refer to the agency's or facility's policy and procedures manual and look up care of the body following death.

Caring for *You!*

7

Just as the team needs to individualize care to meet the needs of dying people they care for, each member of the team needs to personalize self-care strategies.

1. List, mind map, or draw activities that help you to refuel and re-energize.

reflections

2. Reflect on the term "self-care." Write freely for five minutes about the topic of self-care. What did you learn? Where did your reflections take you?

_____

_____

_____

_____

_____

_____

_____

_____

_____

_____

_____

_____

_____

_____

_____

_____

_____

_____

_____

_____

_____

_____

_____

_____

3. Review the information about compassion fatigue in Chapter 7 of the text.

   a. Write freely for five minutes about compassion fatigue.

_____

_____

_____

_____

_____

_____

_____

_____

_____

_____

_____

_____

_____

_____

_____

_____

_____

_____

_____

_____

_____

_____

b. Review the chart on pages 206 and 207 in the text. What zone are you in?

Red   **Green**   **Yellow**   (circle your answer)

c. Respond to the reflection questions in the table on Compassion Fatigue that relate to the zone you are in.

_____

_____

_____

_____

_____

_____

_____

_____

_____

4. Drawing upon the information on pages 210 to 218 of the text, create a maintenance self-care plan using the strategies from each of the categories.

After completing your maintenance self-care plan, meet in pairs or small groups and discuss your self-care plans. Be open to feedback and provide constructive support to your colleagues.

Consider how you will know if your maintenance self-care plan is working for you. When would you want to evaluate this plan and assess its successes? Reflect on whether you are open to trying new strategies if the chosen strategies are not working well. Consider arranging a time to meet with your group in the future to check in with one another about self-care, and to evaluate and adjust your self-care plans as needed.

5. Create an emergency self-care plan. Share this plan with a colleague, describing why the strategies in your plan will be most useful for you in an emergency or crisis situation.

6. Education is one of the finest forms of self-care! The books, movies, and websites listed below are about dying, death, palliative care, and caregiving. They were chosen because they are classics, thought-provoking, or just plain good.

a. Circle titles that interest you.

Albom, M. *Tuesdays with Morrie: An Old Man, a Young Man, and Life's Greatest Lesson.* New York: Random House, 1997.

Buckman, R. *I Don't Know What to Say: How to Help and Support Someone Who Is Dying.* Toronto: Key Porter Books, 2005.

Callanan, M., and P. Kelley. *Final Gifts: Understanding the Special Awareness, Needs, and Communications of the Dying.* Toronto: Bantam Books, 1993.

Joseph, E. *In the Slender Margin: The Intimate Strangeness of Dying.* Toronto: HarperCollins, 2014. (This book is a journey into the land of death and dying seen through the lens of art and the imagination.)

Mathieu, F. *The Compassion Fatigue Workbook.* New York: Routledge, 2012.

O'Rourke, M., and E. Dufour. *Embracing the End of Life: Help for Those Who Accompany the Dying.* Toronto: Novalis, 2012.

Schwalbe, W. *The End of Your Life Book Club*. New York: First Vintage Books, 2012.

b. Circle movies that you want to see.

A Story about Care (15-minute video, available on Vimeo at http://vimeo.com/57786711, or Canadian Virtual Hospice, www.virtualhospice.ca).

Empathy: The Human Connection to Patient Care
(4-minute video, available on YouTube at http://youtu.be/cDDWvj_q-o8)

The Bucket List (2007), Jack Nicholson, Morgan Freeman. Two terminally ill men who meet as patients in a hospital head off with a list of things they want to do before they die.

Wit (2001), Emma Thompson. A professor reassesses her life when she finds out she has terminal ovarian cancer.

Five People You Meet in Heaven (2004), Jon Voight, Ellen Burstyn and Jeff Daniels. Eddie is an 83-year-old war vet working as a maintenance man in an amusement park. When he dies while saving a young girl in harm's way from a falling ride, he enters the afterlife and meets five people who will explain the meaning of his life.

c. Circle websites that you want to explore.

Canadian Hospice Palliative Care Association, www.chpca.net

Canadian Virtual Hospice, www.virtualhospice.ca

Life and Death Matters, www.lifeanddeathmatters.ca

Speak Up: Advance Care Planning in Canada, www.advancecareplanning.ca

The Way Forward: An Integrated Palliative Approach to Care, www.hpcintegration.ca

Your provincial hospice palliative care association

Health Canada: Framework on Palliative Care in Canada,
https://www.canada.ca/en/health-canada/services/health-care-system/reports-publications
/palliative-care/framework-palliative-care-canada.html

Ontario Palliative Care Network, Palliative care competencies for PSWs in Ontario,
https://www.ontariopalliativecarenetwork.ca/en/competencyframework

British Columbia Centre for Palliative Care: Inter-professional Palliative Competency Framework:
Health-care Assistants, https://bc-cpc.ca/cpc/publications/competency-framework/

Health Canada: Medical Assistance in Dying,
https://www.canada.ca/en/health-canada/services/medical-assistance-dying.html

Symptom Framework for PSWs adapted for pain

O	**Onset**	When did the pain begin? Is this new, or has this happened before? Did it start suddenly or slowly?
P	**Provoking/Palliating**	What makes the pain feel better? Worse?
Q	**Quality**	Can you describe the discomfort? How does this symptom affect you?
R	**Region/Radiating**	Where are you feeling the pain?

S	**Severity**	How severe is the pain?
		    0 = no symptom and 10 = the worst imaginable
		    Small, medium, large
		    Mild, moderate, severe

T	**Treatment**	What do you think might be helpful?
U	**Understanding**	What do you think might be happening?
V	**Values**	What are your goals for your pain?
W	**What else?**	What else do you want me to know or do? **For the PSW:** Consider your knowledge of this person—what do you see? What do you believe would be helpful?

S | **SITUATION**
My name is _____.
I need to talk with you about _____.
Concern is a   Person's name
- ❏ Change in person's condition
- ❏ Ongoing issue
- ❏ Safety issue
- ❏ Family issue

Is it a good time to talk now? When?

B | **BACKGROUND**
They are experiencing pain.
Relevant information (Include observations from PPS)

A | **ASSESSMENT**
Symptom
(Record information gathered with the Symptom Framework for PSWs)

Onset	
Provoking/Palliating	
Quality	
Region/Radiating	
Severity	
Treatment	
Understanding	
Values	
What else?	

Other concerns:

R | **REQUEST/RECOMMENDATION**
Can you come and see _____?
What do you recommend that I do now?
What is the plan moving forward?

Instructor's Marking Sheet for the Role-Play Exercises on Pain*

*The group, not individual students, will be marked.

Students in group: _____

Role-Play Exercises (circle role-play question #):   #31   #32

Role-Play	Possible Marks	Comments
Student playing the person in pain	1	
Student playing the person in pain describes it using the information provided	1	
Student playing the PSW uses the Symptom Framework for PSWs	1	
Onset	1	
Provoking/Palliating	1	
Quality	1	
Region/Radiating	1	
Severity	1	
Treatment	1	
Understanding	1	
Values	1	
What else?	1	
Nurse receives a clear and complete report from the PSW.	2	
Record/documentation is clear, concise, and accurately reflects the verbal report.	2	
The reporting is free of judgments and focuses on key information.	2	
The students reflect on their learning experience and how they can apply it in practice.	3	
TOTAL MARKS GIVEN	**/21**	

Instructor's Marking Sheet for the Role-Play Exercises on Pain*

* The group, not individual students, will be marked.

Students in group: _____

Role-Play Exercises (circle role-play question #): #31 #32

Role-Play	Possible Marks	Comments
Student playing the person in pain	1	
Student playing the person in pain describes it using the information provided	1	
Student playing the PSW uses the Symptom Framework for PSWs	1	
Onset	1	
Provoking/Palliating	1	
Quality	1	
Region/Radiating	1	
Severity	1	
Treatment	1	
Understanding	1	
Values	1	
What else?	1	
Nurse receives a clear and complete report from the PSW.	2	
Record/documentation is clear, concise, and accurately reflects the verbal report.	2	
The reporting is free of judgments and focuses on key information.	2	
The students reflect on their learning experience and how they can apply it in practice.	3	
TOTAL MARKS GIVEN	**/21**	

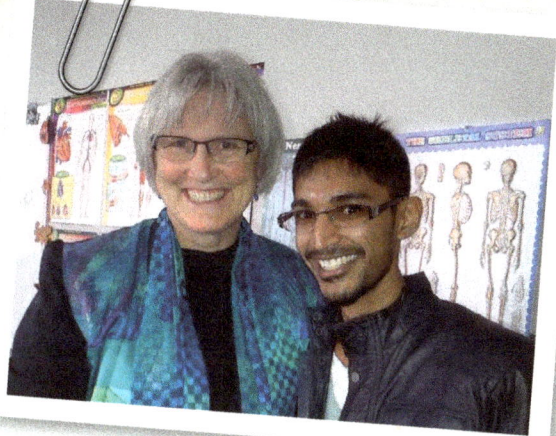

Please feel free to email me your reflections. I so appreciate receiving feedback and stories.

May you feel more comfortable, be more competent, and provide excellent care for the dying and their families. And may your work enrich and bless your life.

Warm regards,
Kath Murray

www.ingramcontent.com/pod-product-compliance
Lightning Source LLC
Chambersburg PA
CBHW050050220326
41599CB00045B/7360